FAMILY & HOMEOWNER'S EARTHQUAKE AND EMERGENCY HANDBOOK

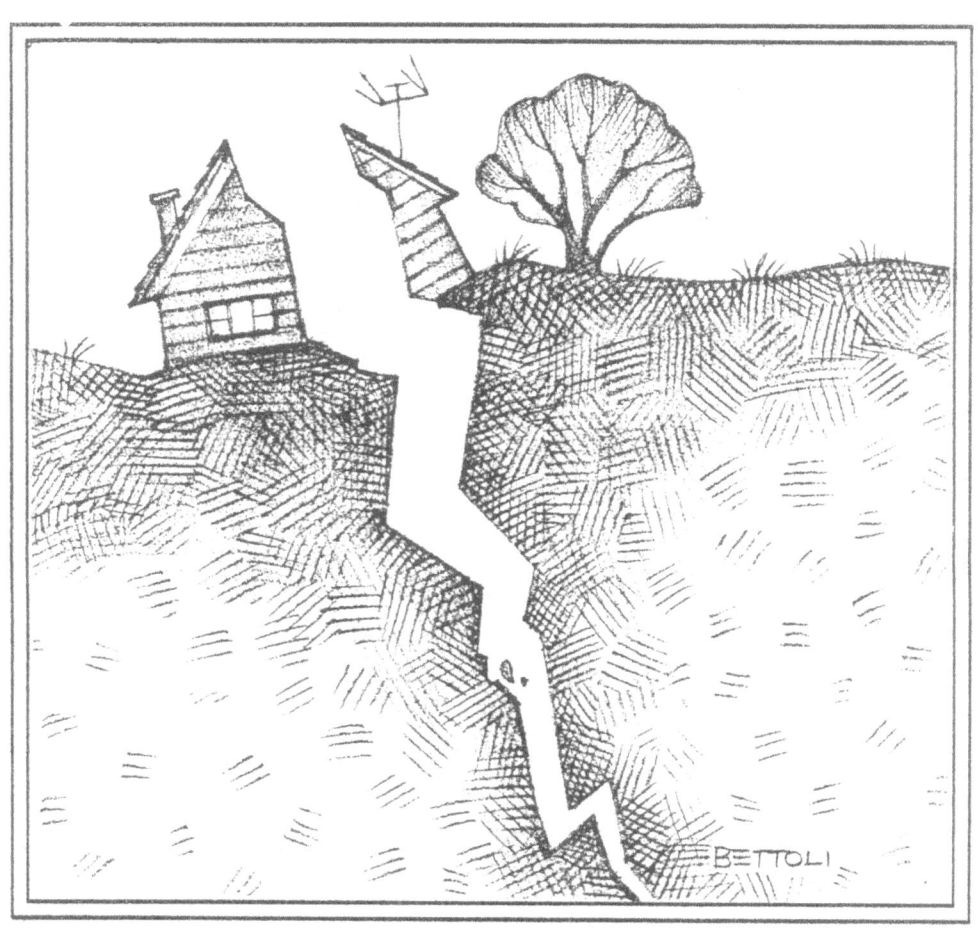

FAMILY & HOMEOWNER'S EARTHQUAKE AND EMERGENCY HANDBOOK

This handbook was compiled from various authoritative sources. The recommendations and suggestions included herein are intended to improve your earthquake, disaster, and emergency awareness and preparedness. While I have tried to insure the accuracy of the information presented here, some of the information may be appropriate for you and your location and some may not be.

The time to read through this handbook is now, long before an emergency presents itself. Fill out the forms, discuss the information with your friends, family, neighbors and co-workers, and adjust the information appropriately, as needed. Most importantly, is the way in which you present these ideas to your minor children. Often, their emotional well being is based on the way in which others around them react to challenging situations. We hope this handbook helps adults present a calm and sensible demeanor before, during, and after a major event. Paranoid and overly obsessive adults, hording caches of supplies and weapons, ready to hunker down or fight off the evil invading masses, will only terrify smaller children and elicit ridicule and distain from older teens and others. Moderation is the key. Find your comfort zone in dealing with preparedness – preferably far from the extremes of neglect and denial on one hand, or hoarding and paranoid hysteria on the other.

INTRODUCTION

<u>GENERAL INFORMATION ABOUT EARTHQUAKES</u>   Earthquakes are a fact of life for people living in California.   Knowledge and preparation are your best tools for effectively dealing with the inevitable "big one." *

Many people try to avoid thinking about earthquakes, either because they are afraid of them or because they doubt that one will ever affect their daily lives.   This is unfortunate. During any serious catastrophe, your survival may depend on how well you cope with emotional stress and shock. The very act of preparing yourself for any calamity can give you the sense of intellectual and physical control critical to lessening stress during and after the event.

Most people spend over half their time at home, which means that you will probably be at home when the major earthquake strikes. That is why we think home preparation is so important.

----

* "The Big One" is really a misleading concept. Don't be too caught up with Richter Scale numbers. We live on a vast network of faults. If, for example, there were a 7.0 event on the Newport Inglewood Fault, it may cause as much damage to homes as an 8.0 event on the San Andreas Fault. Much has to do with location, soil, and other geological conditions.

<u>DEFINING AN EARTHQUAKE</u>   An earthquake, like rain, is a natural phenomenon.   Earthquakes have occurred for billions of years.   Descriptions as old as recorded history show the significant effects they have had on people's lives.   Long before there were scientific theories about the causes of earthquakes, people around the world created folklore to explain them.   In simple terms, earthquakes are caused by the constant motion of the earth's surface.   This motion creates a buildup and a subsequent release of energy that is stored in rocks at and near the surface of the earth.   Earthquakes are the sudden, rapid shaking of the earth as this energy is released.

Earthquakes affect almost every part of the earth.   They can be mild or catastrophic.   Over the course of geological time, earthquakes, floods, and other natural events have helped to shape the surface of our planet.

An earthquake may last only a few seconds, but the dynamics that cause earthquakes have operated within the earth for millions of years. *

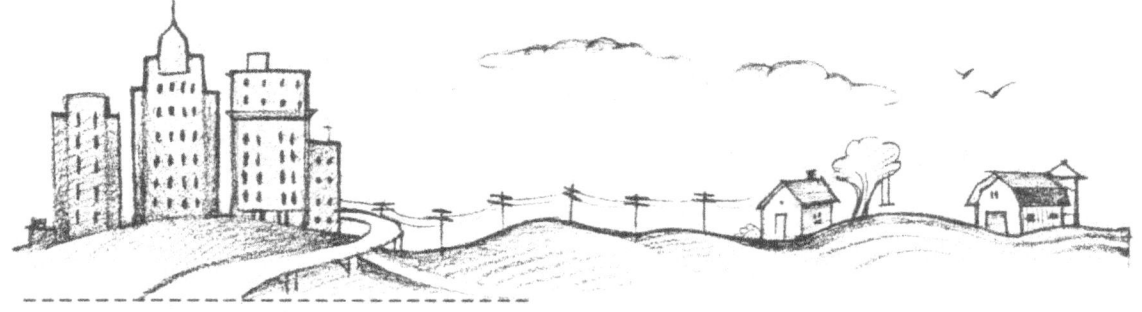

* From <u>EARTHQUAKES,</u> FEMA-159; National Science Teachers Association, October 1988.

PSYCHOLOGICAL CONSIDERATIONS

ADULTS When you are involved in a major earthquake, you will experience severe shaking, you will see buildings damaged beyond repair, and people injured. When these things happen, you may feel that you cannot control your environment or your immediate situation. This can cause psychological stress, which can manifest itself in a variety of ways, including (but not limited to) the following:

Anxiety
Emotional Exhaustion
Confusion
Depression
Aggressive Behavior
Vomiting
Headaches

CHILDREN When adults suffer a traumatic event, such as a major earthquake, they are vulnerable because they have "nothing to do." They often feel that there is something they "should" be doing, but they simply don't know what it is. Children, on the other hand, are usually accustomed to having adults control their environment. More traumatic for many children may be seeing adults out of control. Here are some things to remember in this regard:

1. The tone will be set for many children by the first actions they see adults take.

2. Don't try to tell children that everything is okay when it clearly is not. It is all right to admit

your own fear but at the same time be optimistic.

3. Give children something to do. Letting them participate in <u>some small way</u> will help build their sense of inner control. When they are "working" to help the situation, they are less frightened. Discuss your plans and how your children will be involved. Let them participate in the recovery planning process. Provide structured but undemanding jobs for them to do, depending on their age and physical condition.

4. Be prepared to accept some regressive behavior after this kind of crisis.

5. Children ages four to twelve may cling to adults, or they may become aggressive toward younger siblings. They may not want to be with kids their own age for a while. They may have nightmares, night terrors, or a fear of darkness. They may complain of vague or imagined aches and pains. They may become constipated. Discussing your plan for earthquake preparedness before and after the earthquake will help avoid many serious problems.

6. Older kids may be particularly upset if they cannot return to peer group interactions. It is a good idea to give them an opportunity to help in family or community efforts and then give them a chance to

be with their friends for a while.

7. Have all children participate as best they can in family or community discussions that relive the disaster. Often they will want to demonstrate "what they will do next time." They need to feel that it is okay to have been afraid and to continue to be afraid. It is important that children know that their emotional reactions to the disaster were and are appropriate. It is important that they feel welcome to "talk out their fears" but they should not be forced to do so. Including neighbors or school friends in the discussion may help silent children express themselves.

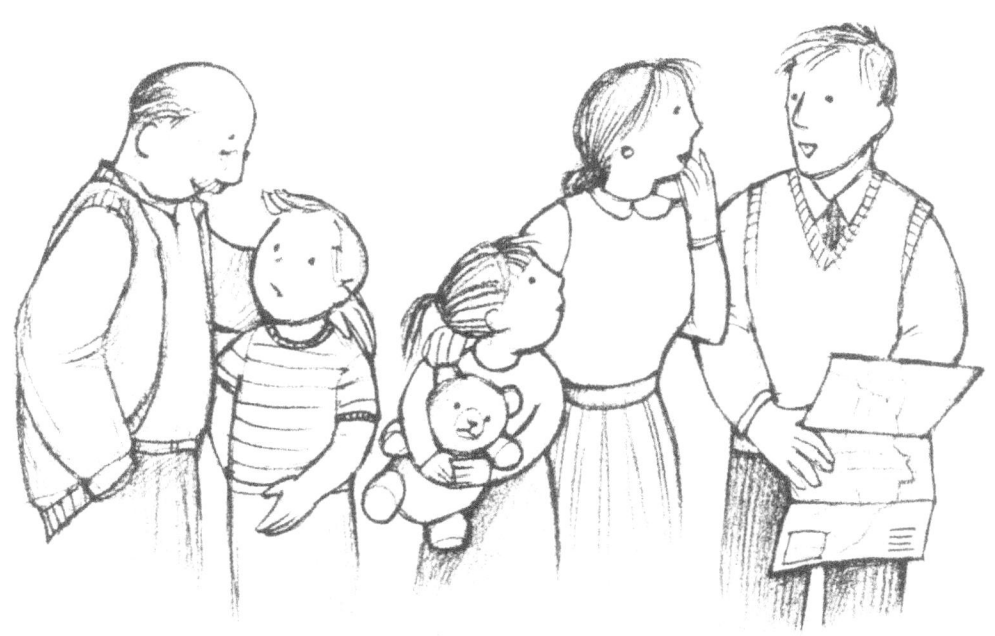

THINGS TO REMEMBER DURING THE SHAKING

REMAIN CALM   Often there will be a noticeable sound right before an earthquake. If you are prepared and have thought about what you would do in an earthquake, the second or two between the sound and the shaking will be enough time for you to react properly automatically. Chances are great that you will do the right thing if you have thought about it in advance. If you remain calm, you will be better able to assess the immediate situation and determine what is the best thing to do.

If you are in a building, stay there. If you think you are in danger, dive under a sturdy table, bed, or desk. Move to an inner wall, away from glass or bookshelves. Things to avoid include china cabinets, sliding glass doors, shower doors, mirrors, and chimneys. If you rush outside you may be injured by falling objects from the roof or exterior structure of your building or of nearby buildings. Also, stairways may be broken and the usual exits may be jammed with people trying to get out. Stay away from elevators, as they may get stuck between floors.

If you are outside, stay there. Move into open spaces, away from buildings, if possible. Avoid lamp posts and power lines. If a power line falls on a chain-link fence, the entire fence could be dangerous. Stay away from anything touching downed power lines, such as damp objects, puddles of water, people lying across the wires, etc. Stay well back!

If you are in a moving car, stop safely and remain in the car. Don't stop on a highway overpass or bridge if you can avoid it. You are usually quite safe in a car out in an open space. On a crowded freeway, you may bounce around quite a bit on the car springs, and you may collide with other vehicles, but you will probably be pretty safe -- a lot safer than you would be trying to walk between the bouncing and colliding cars!

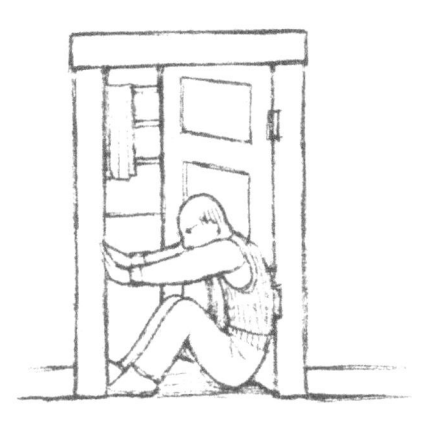
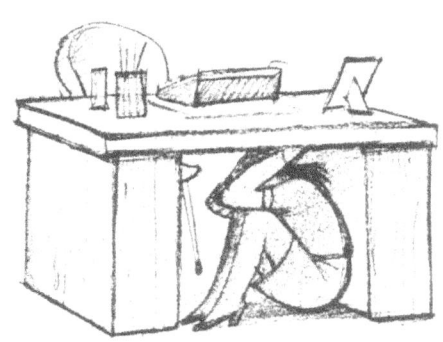

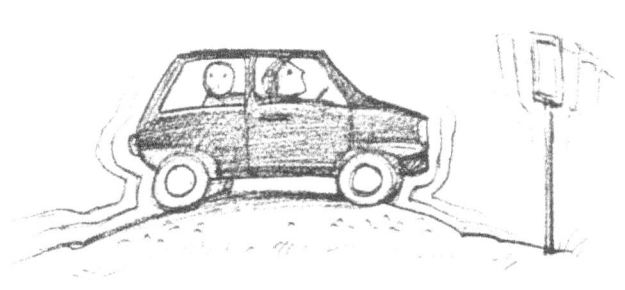
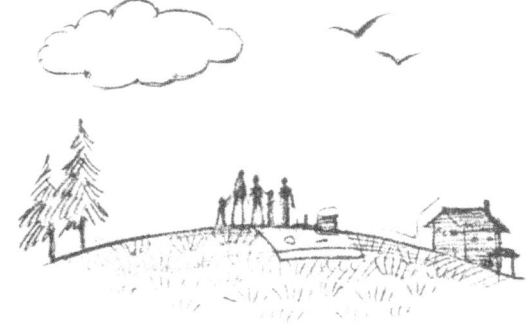

THINGS TO DO FIRST IF YOU ARE AT HOME DURING A QUAKE

1. Don't Panic. Remain Calm. Stay covered and braced until the shaking has stopped completely. Do not run outdoors or downstairs. Aftershocks are almost certain to follow, so don't go into hazardous areas after the earthquake.

2. Put on a good pair of heavy shoes. Keep a pair of shoes and socks under your bed. Cover your head with a newspaper, cardboard box, or blanket if you cannot find a hat or hard hat.

3. Use flashlights for looking around. Don't smoke cigarettes, light matches, or turn on or off electrical switches. If you smell gas, leave immediately.

4. If you DO smell or hear gas, turn off the gas at the meter. If you don't smell or hear gas, don't turn off the gas. Check the stove if you were cooking. Turn off all appliances if you need to focus your attention on earthquake damage.

5. Make a quick check for injured or trapped people. Don't move seriously injured people unless they are in danger of being injured further.

6. Fill your bathtub about half way with cold water.   Use other containers to hold a supply of fresh drinking water, just in case the water service is interrupted.

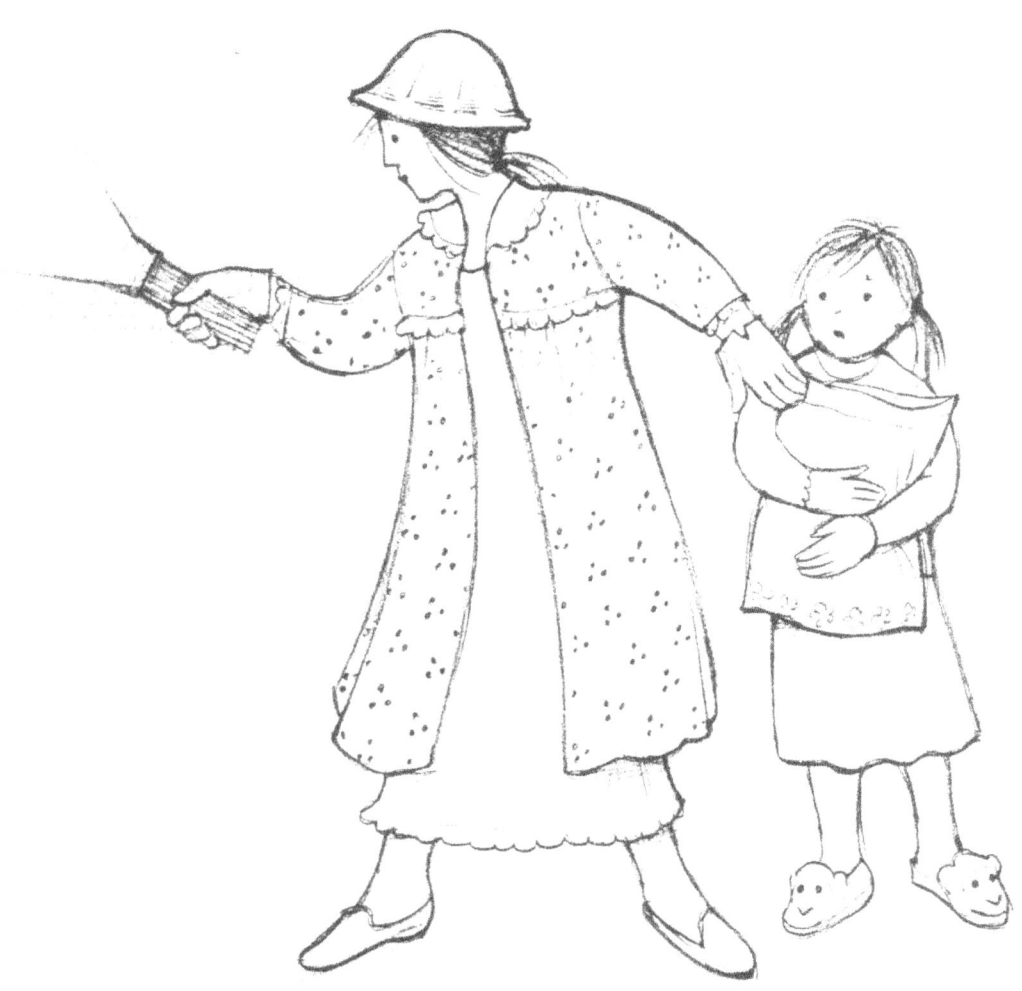

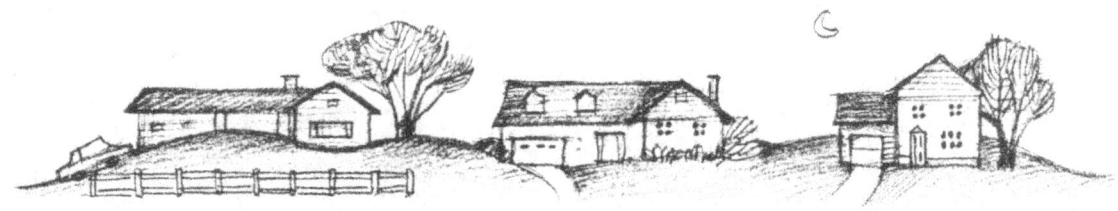

THINGS TO DO A FEW HOURS AFTER THE EARTHQUAKE

1. Take the time to look a little closer at whatever injuries you or people around you may have. Remember, there may be a lot of dirt and dust in the air, and it is important to avoid infections. If you need to free someone who is trapped, remember to carefully remove the debris that is trapping the person <u>piece</u> <u>by</u> <u>piece</u>. Think of the child's game "Pick-Up-Sticks," in which the object is to remove the sticks so carefully that none of the other sticks move.

2. Check your battery operated radio or car radio for any governmental or emergency instructions or information. Don't use the telephone unless it is absolutely essential for you to do so. Even if the telephone service has been knocked out by the earthquake, it is still very important that you replace the telephone receiver on its cradle. When the service comes back on (and this may not be for several days or longer), the system cannot handle all the off-the-hook receivers "requesting" dial tone! Pay phones may work even if other telephone service has been interrupted.

3. Don't drive unless it is absolutely essential. If you must drive, remember to do so very carefully, avoiding emergency vehicles. There may be other people on the road who are less calm than you are, and you will need to be very careful to avoid accidents or confrontations.

4. If practical, clean up any spilled medicines, chemicals, broken glass, etc.

5. Prepare for possible evacuation. Gather the survival supplies listed in this handbook in an easy-to-reach location so you can be prepared to leave at once. Be mindful of secondary emergencies, such as fires, floods, landslides, or tsunamis.

6. Remember to eat food and to drink water so you can maintain your strength and morale. Being sufficiently nourished helps you cope with tough situations. Remind family members to maintain especially high sanitation standards and to keep their fingers out of their mouths.

7. Don't go sightseeing. If you are at home, stay home.

8. If there is a search-and-rescue effort in your area, remember to hang out a white "flag" (sheet, pillow case, towel, undershirt, etc.) to let rescue workers know that you do not require assistance. Try to keep as quiet as possible around rescue areas so searchers can listen more effectively for the sounds of trapped people. Do

not assist in rescue operations unless you have been requested to do so by someone with experience in search and rescue technique.

9. In an extreme emergency, think of your usual civil rights as temporarily suspended. Police, fire, Red Cross, or other emergency personnel may give you orders that, under normal circumstances, might seem unfair or a violation of your rights. If they tell you to leave your home, or that you may not return to your home, or that you may go home but only for an hour, or that you must leave your home before sundown, etc., follow these instructions. Saving lives and preserving property may depend on our ability to follow instructions without arguing.

10. If you evacuate, display your white "flag" and leave a note in a conspicuous place for neighbors or friends, giving your planned destination and route. If you have previously established an out of state contact, as suggested in this handbook, now would be a good time to call them and leave messages, if possible. If you have a cellular phone, check to see if it still works.

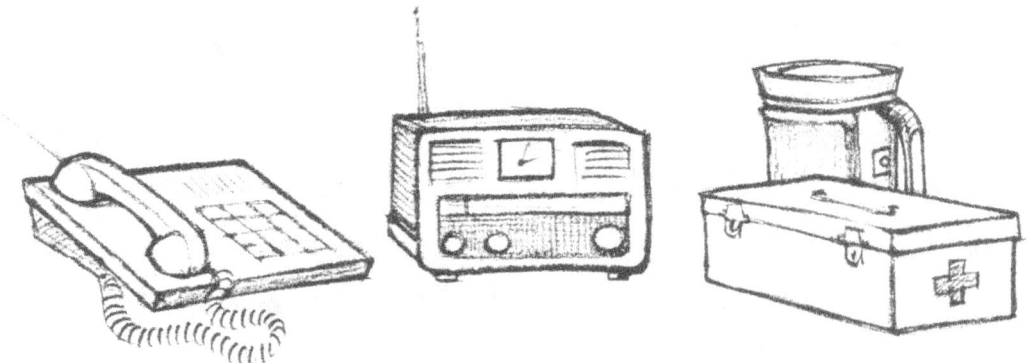

THE FAMILY PLAN

DEVELOP A FAMILY PLAN, ASSIGN RESPONSIBILITIES, AND PRACTICE YOUR PLAN IN ADVANCE. You and your family should develop a good plan for earthquake survival. Each member of your family should have a set of tasks, depending on the situation, and appropriate to their age and skills. Leave nobody out. Even small children (four years and older) can participate in the plan and have their own special emergency duties.

The goal is not merely to have lots of people to do the jobs at hand. Equally important is that everyone feels vitally helpful and part of the team. Keeping people busy with valuable tasks to perform is often very important for their emotional well-being: it is easier to feel strong (and to be strong) when you feel that you are needed. If there are children present, this is especially true for them. This is discussed further in the section on children in this handbook.

Imagine various living condition contingencies: that your house has some damage; that your house is severely damaged and unsafe for occupancy; or that your house and the entire neighborhood are unsafe and that you must evacuate. In the first contingency, you may plan merely to stay home and clean up as best you can. In the second scenario, you may expect to "camp out" in your back yard. In the third situation, you may need to leave your house for an extended

period -- three weeks or longer. Each of these three
conditions requires a different plan.

Document your family plan Put the details of your plan
on paper, so everyone can better visualize his own part of
the whole. You may wish to sketch out a floor plan of your
home, showing secondary exists, location of emergency
supplies or equipment, utility shut-off locations and tools
needed for shut-off operations, etc. Your plan may show a
nearby outside meeting place in case your home is totally
destroyed. Your plan should show the safest place to be in
each room in your house. Take your plan-on-paper sketch and
walk the family through it. Practice getting under tables
and holding on. List your own DO's and DON'Ts on the plan.

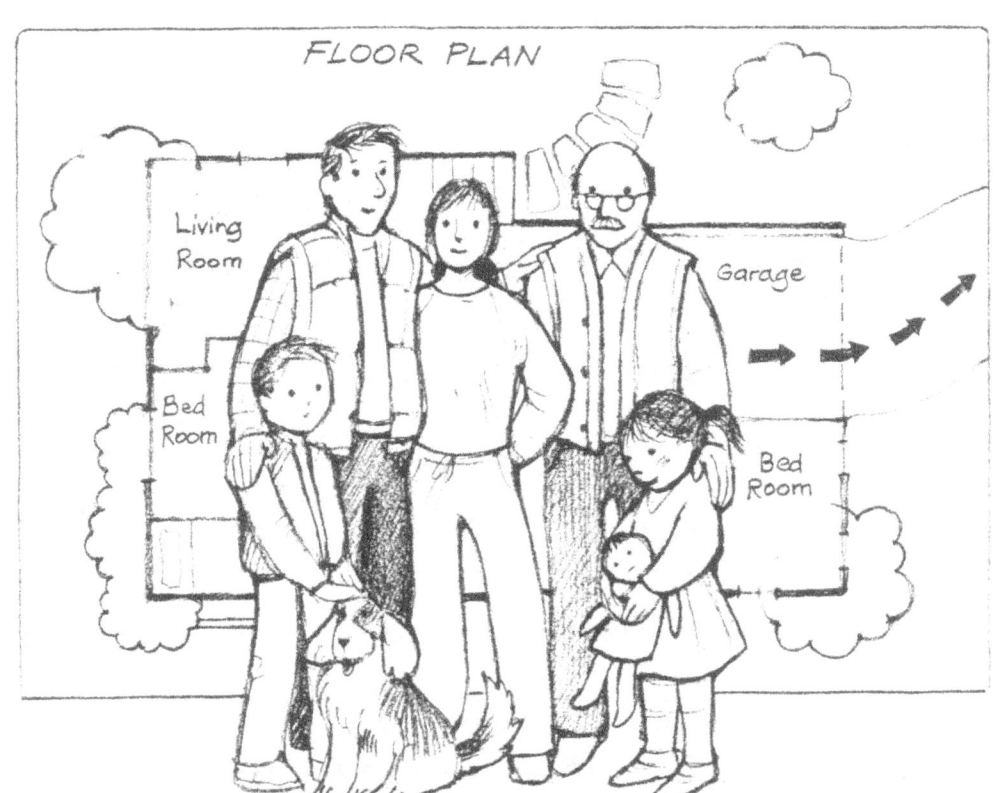

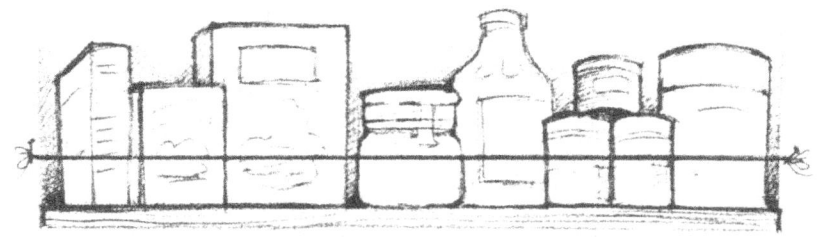

SUPPLIES

First a word of caution. Many people get carried away with the idea of "survival supplies." This may be a holdover from the days of civil defense and bomb shelters, when many people would hoard huge quantities of food, ready to "lock and load" their weapons to fend off desperate neighbors panicking as the fallout began to rain down on them. As a result, many people subconsciously and mistakenly associate preparedness with paranoia and planning with reactionary politics.

Not all of the supplies listed in this handbook are essential. As a matter of fact, except for a little food and water, there is very little that you really need to survive. There are, however, many "What if..." situations in which many of the items found on the following pages would be greatly appreciated and beneficial, if not absolutely essential. Please feel free to pick and chose. It is up to you how much of your life you want to dedicate to disaster preparedness. Whatever you decide to do, remember to keep your supplies where you could get to them after an earthquake. Don't keep them in your garage, for example, since garages tend to be structurally weaker than other parts of the house.

Most important, of course, is the plan. Psychological

preparation is a valuable by-product of the process of formulating some kind of plan. A plan for family communication is paramount. The items listed below could be extremely important in <u>some</u> situations; none of them is essential in <u>all</u> situations.

Besides the usual list of first-aid supplies and emergency equipment, most of the items included serve to keep the situation more manageable or comfortable. For example, we list hard candy as something to keep in the emergency kits. Besides helping to put a smile on a face, the sugar in hard candies or chewing gum helps keep electrolytes in your body; electrolytes are essential to maintaining health and energy. Nobody will die without toilet paper either, but for some people this added convenience is greatly appreciated when everything else around them seems to be chaotic.

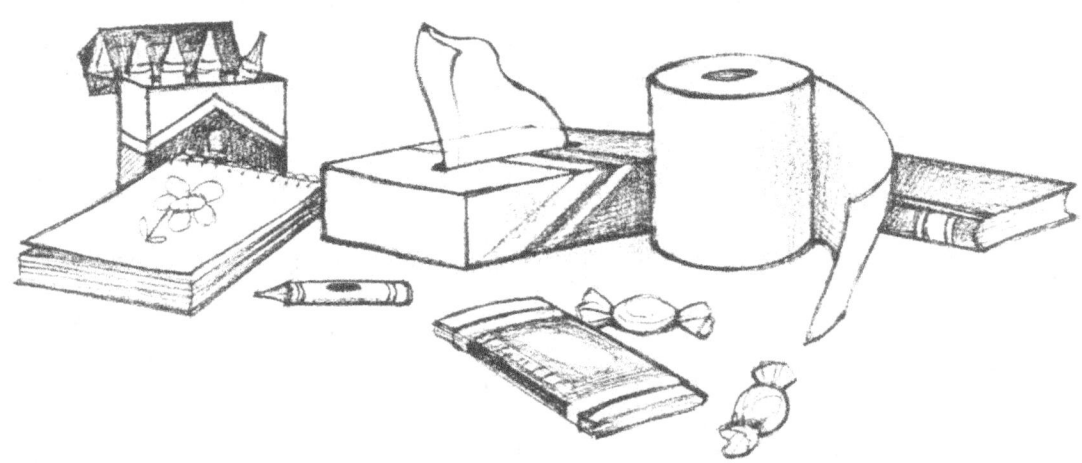

On the following pages, a rather extensive list of items you may wish to purchase is divided into different sections, as follows:

FIRST AID SUPPLIES
DISASTER PREPAREDNESS KIT
THE SIX-WEEK SHOPPING LIST *

Many items are repeated on each list, particularly first-aid supplies. Each list represents a different approach to deciding what you may need in case of a major earthquake. Remember that all these supplies are no substitute for what is <u>really</u> important -- taking the time to prepare a PLAN for yourself and for your family. After a major quake, don't expect to get any help for an extended period. Being self-reliant is really the key!

---

* The Six Week Shopping List is taken from <u>Living With Our Faults: An Earthquake Survival Guide,</u> Published by the Regents of the University of California. The Six-Week Shopping List was designed to spread out your initial earthquake preparedness shopping over a period of time, so that it does not disrupt your family budget too much. Also, buying too much all at once may be overwhelming. It is much better to take the time and really decide what you want to purchase and how it fits into your overall plan.

FIRST-AID KIT

Drugs
Prescribed medications
Photocopies of prescriptions
Antibiotic ointment
Aspirin and nonaspirin
Diarrhea medication
Laxative
Eye drops
Antiseptic wash
Ipecac syrup
Nose drops and ear drops
Cough medicine
Benadryl

Dressings
Band-Aids
Ace bandages
Gauze pads
Adhesive tape roll
Triangular bandage
   (37" X 37")
Sterile eye pads
Butterfly bandages
Cotton swabs and Q-Tips
Sterile roll bandage
   (2" wide)
Duct tape
Clean sheets to cut into
   strips for slings
Dust masks
First-aid book
Saline solution

Other Supplies
Tweezers
Scissors
Safety pins
Liquid Bleach
Razor Blades
Soap
Sanitary Napkins
Needles, thread
Pocket knife
Plastic spoons
Skin cream
Vaseline
Kleenex
Thermometer
Baking Soda
Coarse Salt
Dental floss
Hydrogen peroxide
Chemical hot packs
Chemical cold packs
Insect repellent
Paper, pen, pencil
Rubbing alcohol
Calamine lotion
Sunscreen lotion
Paper cups
Space blanket
Wooden matches
Medicine dropper
Emergency telephone
   numbers and lots
   of quarters

THE SEARS DISASTER PREPAREDNESS KIT

This kit is designed to meet your immediate needs when a major disaster strikes. It can be used in schools, office buildings, public buildings, apartment complexes, condominium complexes, malls, or factories. All of the items below fit inside a mobile container and are available from Sears.

FOUR MAN (Person) TEAM
 4 Hard hats
12 Prs. leather palmed gloves
 4 Eye guards
12 Dust masks
 4 Flashlights and batteries
 4 Safety vests
 4 Whistles
 4 Grease markers
 8 Lightsticks (12-hours each)

ENTRY AND DEBRIS REMOVAL TOOLS
Shovel 27" D-grip Square and round point
Fire axe, 6 pounds
Hacksaw and blades
Wrecking bar, 30 inches
Jack, 6-ton hydraulic
Trash can on wheels (30 Gallon)
Rope, 1/2 inch X 100 feet

EMERGENCY HAND TOOLS
Pipe wrench, 14 inches
Adjustable wrench 10 inches
Screwdriver set, 4 piece
Plier set, 3 piece
Hammer, claw type
Knife, electrician's

OTHER ITEMS
Saline solution
Adhesive tape
Adhesive bandages
Multi trauma Pads
Gauze pads
Instant ice packs
Smelling salts
Assorted bandages
Eye pads
Scissors
Tweezers
Penlight
Tensor bandage
Antiseptic wipes
Antiseptic cream
Tourniquet
Arm splints
Gauze sponges
Nonaspirin
First-aid book
Tongue depressors
Gloves
Space blankets
Solar blankets
Water tablets

SIX-WEEK SHOPPING LIST

Check off items as you purchase them.

WEEK ONE

MARKET

_____2 1/2 Gallons water per person
_____Hand operated can opener
_____Powdered milk
_____1 large jar peanut butter per person
_____Canned juice
_____Canned meat (or tuna)
_____Canned fruit
_____Canned vegetables
_____Baby food
_____Instant coffee, tea, cocoa
_____Powdered cream

HARDWARE STORE

_____Short handled crescent wrench
_____A-B-C type fire extinguishers
_____Crowbar
_____Saw
_____Shovel
_____Axe
_____Broom
_____Dust pan
_____Heavy rope
_____Water turn-off key
_____Plumber's tape
_____Chemical lightsticks
_____Flashlights (2 per person)

WEEK TWO

DRUG STORE

_____ Complete first-aid guide book
_____ Scissors, tweezers
_____ Single-edge razor blades
_____ Aspirin and nonaspirin
_____ Antihistamines
_____ Pepto Bismal
_____ Band-Aids
_____ Compressors
_____ Butterfly bandages
_____ Sterile 4" x 4" gauze pads
_____ Rolls of gauze bandages
_____ Rolls of sterile cotton

MARKET

_____ 2 1/2 gallons of water per person
_____ 1 package paper plates per person
_____ 1 package plastic flatware per person
_____ 25 paper cups (hot and cold) per person
_____ Paper towels
_____ Kleenex
_____ Sanitary napkins (for first aid as well
        as for feminine hygiene)
_____ 4 rolls toilet paper per person
_____ Disposable diapers (for first aid as well
        as for infant needs)
_____ Ziplock plastic bags -- small and large
_____ 3 packages plastic wrap
_____ 3 packages heavy duty aluminum foil

WEEK THREE

MISCELLANEOUS

Evacuation items such as
_____ Sleeping bags
_____ Tent(s)
_____ Portable toilet
_____ Water purification
       Tablets

_____ One case each of paper
      towels and toilet
      paper for barter as
      as for personal use

_____ One large roll of heavy
      gauge plastic to cover
      shattered windows or
      doors

MARKET

_____ Assorted Tupperware
_____ Sponges
_____ Wooden stir spoons
_____ Safety pins
_____ Pencils, pens
_____ Notepads
_____ Charcoal
_____ Q-Tips
_____ Cotton puffs
_____ Hand lotion
_____ Vaseline

HARDWARE

_____ Extra batteries and bulbs
_____ Portable AM radio(s)
_____ Camping lantern
_____ Hammer, nails
_____ Screwdriver
_____ Pliers
_____ Heavy duty work gloves
_____ Masking tape
_____ Duct tape
_____ Extra heavy duty trash bags
      to be used to "bag the toilet" --
      put a bag in toilet bowl over
      the rim, under the seat; tie
      off and replace with fresh bag
      daily

WEEK FOUR

DRUG STORE

_____ Ace bandages
_____ Cotton swabs
_____ Adhesive tape
_____ Large triangular bandages
_____ Tongue depressors
_____ Thermometer
_____ Topical antibiotic ointment
_____ Nausea medicine
_____ Diarrhea medicine
_____ Laxative
_____ Ipecac syrup
_____ Aerosol (or pump) burn spray
_____ Smelling salts
_____ Insect bite medicine
_____ Insect repellent
_____ Rubbing alcohol
_____ Hydrogen peroxide
_____ Antiseptic soap
_____ Chemical hot packs
_____ Chemical cold packs
_____ Vitamin C, chewable or powder

MARKET

Quick energy snacks such as
_____ Granola bars
_____ Raisins
_____ Beef or chicken jerky
_____ Nuts
_____ Candy
_____ Chewing gum
_____ Graham crackers
_____ Dry cereals
_____ Honey

WEEK FIVE

MARKET

____Sun block
____Sun screen
____Toothpaste
____Toothbrushes
____Mild liquid soap
____Deodorant
____Disinfectant
____Baking soda

MISCELLANEOUS

____ At least $100 cash
____ One roll quarters
____ One roll dimes
____ Extra eye glasses
____ Hearing aid batteries
____ Copies of prescriptions
____ Liquid bleach for
     water purification

WEEK SIX

HARDWARE STORE

_____Plastic drop cloths
_____Camping knife
_____Waterproof matches
_____Plastic cigarette lighter
_____Camp stove, BBQ, or hibachi
_____Starter for cooking apparatus
_____Fuel or charcoal for cooking apparatus
_____Powdered chlorinated lime
_____Long lasting candles
_____Angle brackets, screw eye hooks,
      twine, safety latches, plastic bags
      to put in toilet bowl when water
      is unavailable

EMERGENCY CLOTHING

Keep the following items handy:

Shoes, comfortable but must be closed heels and toes
Layered Clothing, cotton and wool
Levis, or other sturdy canvas-type pants
Hats, hard hat and watch cap
Parka, with a hood
Gloves, sturdy and warm
Jacket, warm and water-tight
Boots, broken-in and comfortable

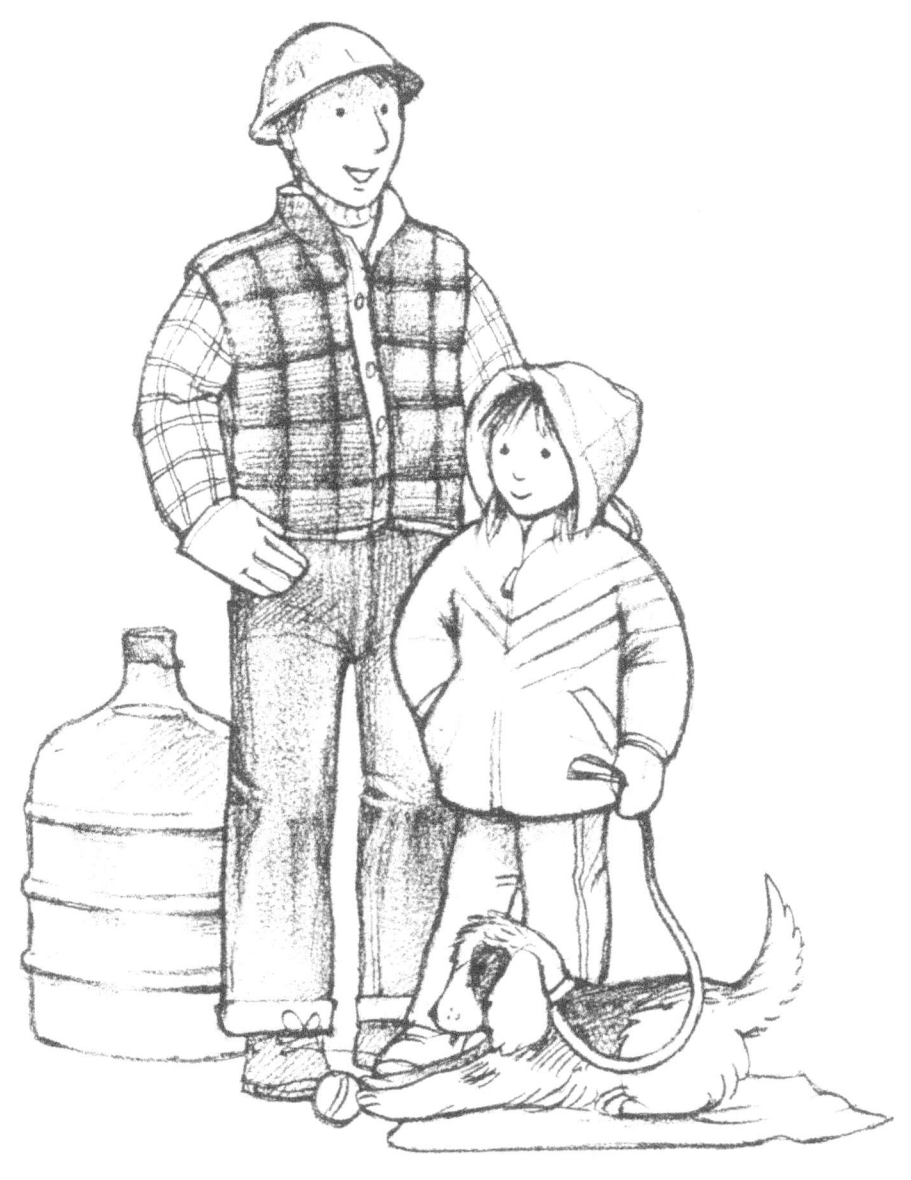

WATER

We can endure many things, but we cannot live without water. The average person should drink at least two quarts of water a day. A gallon per day is preferable, if it is available. A family of four would really require a minimum of approximately 15 gallons of pure drinking water per week. It is also nice to have water for cleaning. While we should not drink swimming pool water, we can certainly use this water for nondrinking purposes. For sanitation reasons, however, even this water must be controlled to ensure its continued cleanliness.

Often you can find good drinking water in a number of places around the home. Water drained from your hot water heater is the most obvious example. To draw water from your hot water heater, turn off the gas or electricity supply, disconnect or open the valve at the top of the heater to let air in, close the inlet-water valve, and then open the bottom faucet to get water. Drain the water into containers. Remember that water is heavy; it is better to make many trips with smaller containers than hurt yourself trying to carry too large a container. After things are back to normal, be sure the water heater is properly connected and full of water before turning the gas or electricity back on.

You can also find water in your household plumbing. Gravity will cause the water to flow down to the lowest valve around your home, even after the water is turned off. Open a faucet on the top floor and drain water from the faucet at the lowest point in your home. You can also drink water from the flush tank (not from the bowl) of your toilets, provided you do not put water-coloring devices or other chemicals in this tank. You can get drinking liquid from melted ice cubes, canned fruit, vegetable juices, and other canned food products.

You can sterilize bottles by washing them in soapy water and rinsing them thoroughly. Then fill the container about half way with whatever washing or cleaning water you have available. Add 1/4 cup liquid bleach for each container quart you have. REMEMBER: this bleach-and-water solution is for sterilizing and is not fit for drinking! Shake the contents well. Let the solution stand for five minutes or so. Turn the container upside down a few times to be sure the cap or lid also comes into contact with the sterilizing solution. Then pour your chlorine disinfecting liquid into your next container for sterilization. Be sure you emptied the liquid from your now clean container. Fill the container with pure drinking water and label it DRINKING WATER -- PURIFIED.

To purify water, use the following formulas:

AMOUNT OF WATER	AMOUNT OF CHLORINE BLEACH TO ADD TO:	
	Clear water	Cloudy water
1 quart	2 drops	4 drops
1 gallon	8 drops	12 drops
5 gallons	1/2 teasp	1 teasp

AMOUNT OF WATER	AMOUNT OF 2 PERCENT TINCTURE OF IODINE TO ADD TO:	
	Clear water	Cloudy water
1 quart	4 drops	6 drops
1 gallon	12 drops	24 drops
5 gallons	3/4 teasp	1 1/2 teasp

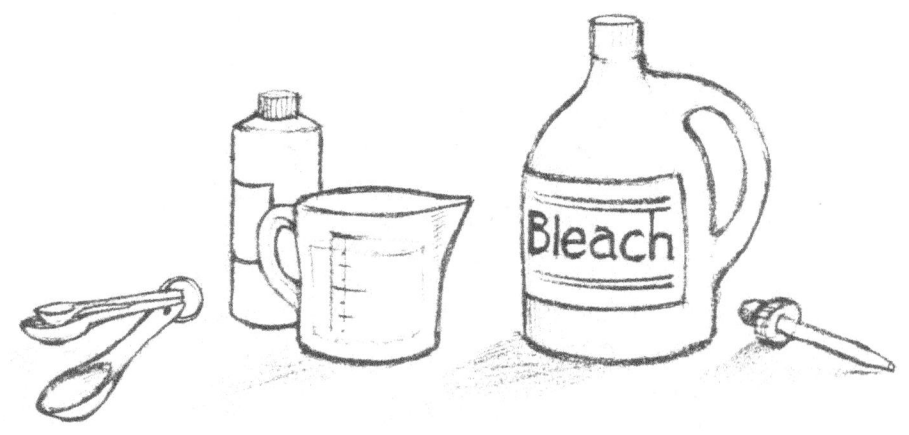

HOME CHECKLIST

_____ 1. Place beds so that they are not next to large windows

_____ 2. Place beds so that they are not right below hanging lights

_____ 3. Place beds so that they are not right below heavy mirrors

_____ 4. Place beds so that they are not right below framed pictures

_____ 5. Place beds so that they are not right below shelves with lots of things that can fall

_____ 6. Replace heavy lamps on bed tables with light, nonbreakable lamps

_____ 7. Change hanging plants from heavy pots into lighter pots

_____ 8. Use closed hooks on hanging plants, lamps

_____ 9. Make sure hooks are attached to studs

_____ 10. Remove heavy objects from high shelves

_____ 11. Remove breakable things from high shelves

_____ 12. Replace latches, such as magnetic touch latches on cabinets, with latches that will hold during an earthquake

_____ 13. Take glass bottles out of medicine cabinet and put them on lower shelves. If there are small children around, make sure you use childproof latches when you move things to lower shelves

_____ 14. Remove glass containers that are around the bathtub

_____ 15. Move materials that can easily catch fire so that they are not close to heat sources

_____ 16. Attach water heater to the studs of the nearest wall

_____ 17. Move heavy objects away from exit routes in your house

_____ 18. Block wheeled objects so that they cannot roll

_____ 19. Attach tall heavy furniture such as bookshelves to studs in the walls

_____ 20. Use flexible connectors where gas lines meet appliances such as stoves, water heaters, and clothes dryers

_____ 21. Attach heavy appliances such as refrigerators to studs in the walls

_____ 22. If you have a brick chimney, nail plywood to ceiling joists to protect people from chimney bricks that could fall through the ceiling

_____ 23. Make sure heavy mirrors are well fastened to walls

_____ 24. Make sure heavy pictures are well fastened to walls

_____ 25. Make sure air conditioners are well braced

_____ 26. Make sure all roof tiles are secure

_____ 27. Brace outside chimney, if any

_____ 28. If you have a single-family residence, bolt the house to the foundation (you may want to have this professionally done)

_____ 29. Remove dead or diseased tree limbs that could fall on your house

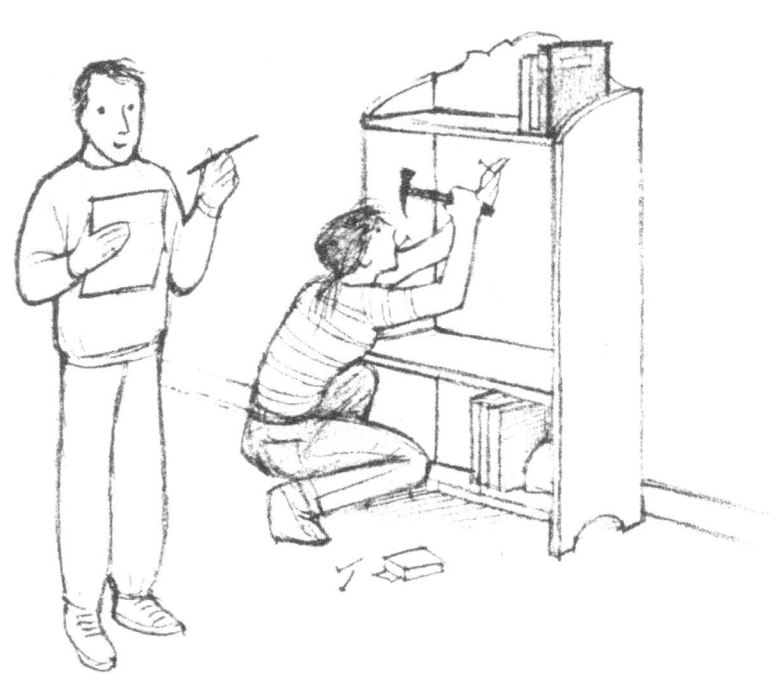

ONE MONTH FOOD SUPPLY FOR A BALANCED DIET

Type of Food	Amount Per Person	Notes
MILK	14 QUARTS	One quart of milk is equal to four ounces dry milk.
CHEESE	3 POUNDS	
TUNA OR OTHER CANNED MEATS EGGS BEANS NUTS, etc.	16 POUNDS (60 servings)	One serving could be 3 oz. meat, poultry or fish; or two eggs; or one cup cooked dried beans; or 1/2 cup nuts; or five tablespoons of peanut butter.
FRUITS VEGETABLES JUICES	15 POUNDS plus FOUR 46 OZ CANS OF FRUIT JUICES OR V-8 JUICE	One service is either four ounces of canned fruit or vegetables or two ounces of dried fruit or eight ounces canned juice.
FATS and COOKING OILS	TWO POUNDS	Use kinds that require no refrigeration.
SUGAR	HALF POUND	
SALT	HALF POUND	
FLOUR	TWO POUNDS	
CANDIES HONEY MOLASSES PUDDINGS JAM, etc.	FOUR POUNDS	

Some foods can be stored longer than others. Below is a list of some groups of foods that can be stored for emergency use; note their suggested replacement periods. These foods should be "rotated" (used and replaced with fresh foods) into your usual family diet. Remember, buy foods sensibly. Do not hoard large quantities of foods. To do so is not only selfish, but usually results in waste and improperly balanced meals. Remember, in the event of an emergency where the power goes off, use the food in your refrigerator first. Next use the food in your freezer. Then start on your supply of nonperishable foods. Please note that the rotate-and-replace dates are short. This does not necessarily mean that food you keep longer is not wholesome. It only means that we suggest rotating these foods to maintain freshness.

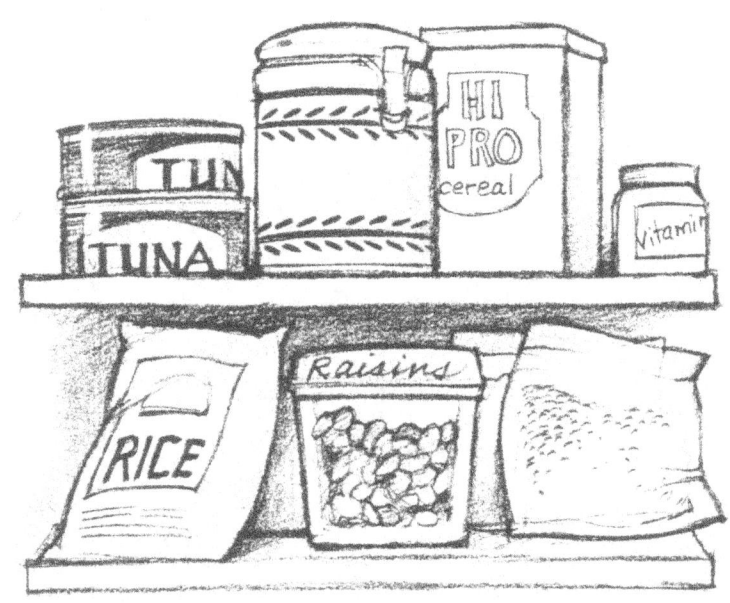

ROTATE OR REPLACE

Every four months:

    Vegetable Oils
    Ready-to-eat Cereals that have been kept sealed
    Brown or Powdered Sugar

Every six months:

    Evaporated Milk
    Nonfat dry or whole dry milk, in metal container
    Pancake mix in airtight container
    Rice mixes
    Instant breakfast liquids and bars

Every nine months:

    Unopened peanut butter

Every twelve months:

    Canned fish (tuna, etc.)
    Meat and vegetable soups
    Canned nuts
    Canned berries, sour cherries, citrus juices
    Canned tomatos, sauerkraut
    Ready-to-eat cereals in metal container
    Uncooked cereal in original container
    Hydrogenated solid shortening
    Honey, jams, syrups kept tightly covered
    Pudding mixes
    Bouillon products that have been kept dry
    Flour (all kinds) kept in airtight container
    Baking soda

Every eighteen months:

    Canned meat or poultry
    Mixtures of meat, vegetables, cereal products
    Non-citrus fruit juices
    Instant potatoes
    Dry beans, dry peas, most canned vegetables
    Instant coffee, cocoa

Every twenty-four months:
    Uncooked cereals in metal container
    Pasta kept in airtight container
    White rice kept in airtight container

Indefinite, kept in an airtight container:
    Salt
    Granulated sugar

REMEMBER -- THE BEST STORAGE PLACES ARE COOL, DRY, AND DARK.

You might want to make a note on your calendar to rotate food and other supplies (medicines, batteries, etc.), since we often tend to forget these things without little reminders.

Immediately following a major earthquake somewhere in the world, people get serious about earthquake preparedness. But soon afterwards, interest diminishes very rapidly.

Since the next major quake may happen tonight or it may not happen for years, preparedness cannot be a one-time event. Instead, it must be a continuing process. It does not have to take much time or cost a lot of money. All that is really required is a little common sense, some planning, and some handy supplies.

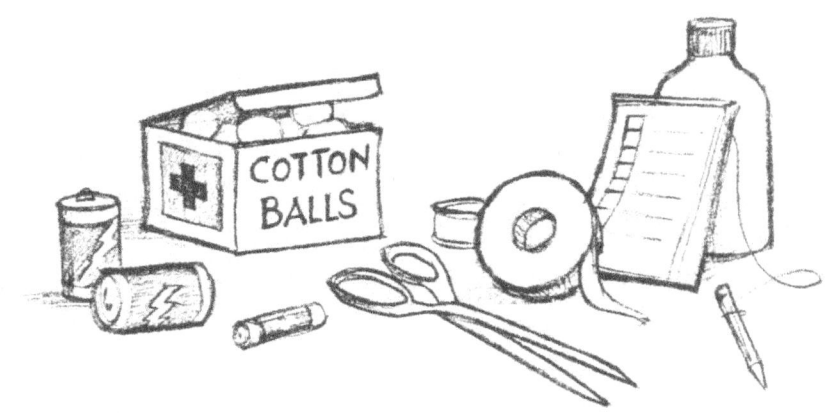

EVACUATION NOTE

I have gone to _____

_____ at _____ (time)

on _____ (date).

I plan to take the following route to get there:

_____

_____

_____

_____

My emergency contact's name is : _____

Their telephone number is: _____
                                  (AREA CODE)   NUMBER

I will try to make contact at _____ (time)
and I will periodically try to make contact after that.

This is a summary of the information I have: _____

_____

_____

_____

I request that you _____

_____

_____

_____

Signed: _____   Dated: _____

SAMPLE INFORMATION FORMS

Feel free to photocopy (on hard card stock if you like) any of the forms in this book. You may wish to design your own

forms or use the sample forms below.

Out of State
Emergency Contact

Name:_____
Address:_____
_____
Phone (W):_____
Phone (H):_____
Husband Work #_____
Wife Work #_____
Kids School #_____

LOCAL
EMERGENCY CONTACT

Name:_____
Address:_____
_____
Phone:_____
Phone:_____

EMERGENCY INFORMATION FOR CHILD

NAME: _____
ADDRESS: _____
_____
HOME PHONE: _____
DATE OF BIRTH: _____
MOM'S PHONE: _____
DAD'S PHONE: _____
NAME OF OUT-OF-STATE CONTACT:
_____
OUT-OF-STATE PHONE: _____

Although this form makes reference to California, most other places will accept this language, particularly in an emergency. Remember that each child needs a separate copy at each school, doctor's office, hospital, babysitter, etc. You should keep a copy in your family emergency-preparedness file. Keep a list of location on file as well, in case you need to make changes on all of the copies.

MEDICAL CARE AUTHORIZATION

Pursuant to *California Family Code* §6910, I, _____, a parent having legal custody of _____, a minor child, hereby authorize _____, an adult person into whose care such minor child has been entrusted, to consent to any X-ray examination (or similar examination such as by CAT scan, MRI, etc.), anesthetic, medical or surgical diagnosis or treatment and hospital care to be rendered to the minor under the general or special supervision and upon the advice of a physician and surgeon licensed under the provisions of the Medical Practice Act or other pertinent Act, or to consent to an X-ray examination, anesthetic, dental or surgical diagnosis or treatment and hospital care to be rendered to the minor by a dentist licensed under the provisions of the Dental Practice Act or other pertinent Act. I agree to pay any and all costs for the foregoing. My medical insurance provider is _____ and my insurance certificate number and/or group number is _____.

Dated:_____

Signed:_____

FOR PATIENT'S PROTECTION

1. __Allergies__ __and__ __sensitivities:__ Is there a history of skin reaction or other adverse reaction or sickness following injection or oral administration of any of the following?

                                                    Circle
                                                     One

PENICILLIN OR OTHER ANTIBIOTICS	YES	NO
MORPHINE, CODEINE, DEMEROL, ETC.	YES	NO
NOVACAINE OR OTHER ANESTHETICS	YES	NO
ASPIRIN, EMPERIN, PAIN REMEDIES	YES	NO
SULFA DRUGS	YES	NO
TETANUS ANTITOXIN OR OTHER SERUMS	YES	NO
ADHESIVE TAPE	YES	NO
IODINE OR MERTHIOLATE	YES	NO
OTHER MEDICATIONS, FOODS, OR DRUGS	YES	NO

    If yes, describe below:

_____

_____

_____ .

2. Has the patient ever received treatment for asthma, rheumatism, or rheumatic fever?   YES   NO

3. Drugs taken by patient within the past six months:

CORTISONE	YES	NO
ACTH	YES	NO
ANTICOAGULANTS	YES	NO
TRANQUILIZERS	YES	NO
HYPOTENSIVES	YES	NO

Other important medical information:

_____

_____

_____

_____

_____   _____

Signature of person acquiring this information   Date

Noted by: _____, M.D.

Every family member should have an emergency-contact information sheet or card with them at all times. Adults and older children should memorize the out-of-state emergency telephone number. Be sure that your children's school, church, babysitter, grandparents, etc. all know about the out-of-state contact. Keep this information in your car, at your place of work, and at a friend's house as well as at home. Just having the information "on file" at school, for example, may not be sufficient. It is also good to have a card or sheet laminated so that it can stay in your children's lunch pails or book bags.

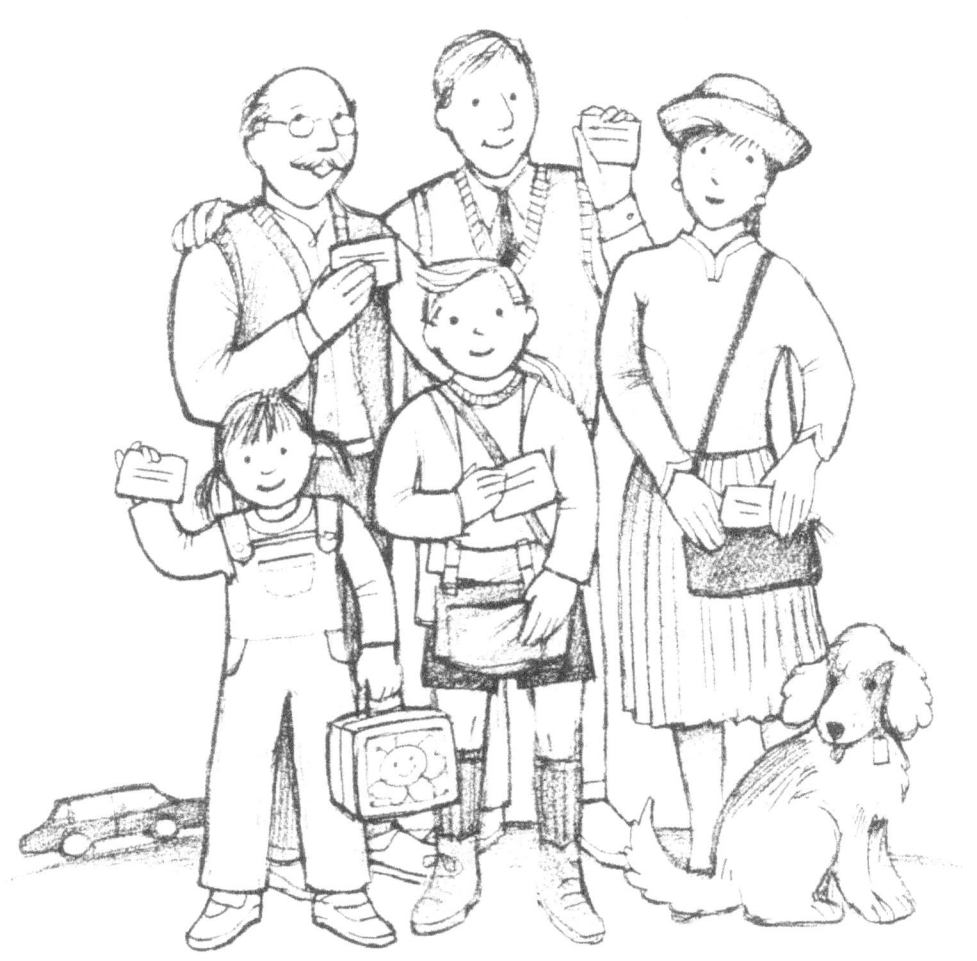

It almost goes without saying, but I'll say it anyway: the time to visit these web sites is before an earthquake or other disaster or emergency – when you have the time to read, learn, and prepare, and when you have power and Internet access!

Links to additional information and supplies

http://www.ready.gov/ and http://www.ready.gov/earthquakes/

http://www.fema.gov/library/viewRecord.do?id=1449

http://www.scouting.org/scoutsource/Media/Publications/EmergencyPreparedness.aspx

http://www.quakekare.com/emergency-supplies-kits/recommended-preparedness-kits.html

http://www.seismic.ca.gov/pub/CSSC%2009-03%20The%20Study%20of%20Household%20Preparedness.pdf

http://www.calema.ca.gov/Pages/default.aspx and http://www.calema.ca.gov/PlanningandPreparedness/Pages/Earthquakes-and-Tsunamis.aspx

http://72hours.org/

http://mitigation.eeri.org/

http://www.costco.com/Service/FeaturePage.aspx?ProductNo=11659938

http://www.homedepot.com/h_d1/N-5yc1v/Ntk-Extended/Ntt-Emergency%2BPreparedness%2BKits/h_d2/Navigation?langId=-1&storeId=10051&catalogId=10053

http://www.walmart.com/catalog/product.do?product_id=10927662&adid=bzv_fb_revshr_001

http://www.thereadystore.com/survival-kits/deluxe-all-in-one-survival-kit-4-person/?aid=4b9e38954d106

http://www.urbachletter.com/0306/ComprehensiveChecklist.htm